Hair Gone Wild!

Recipes & Remedies

for Natural Tresses

Hair Gone Wild!
Recipes & Remedies for Natural Tresses

Printed in the United States of America
ISBN: 978-0-9839155-6-0

Cover Design by: Diane Kidman

Published by: carp(e) libris press, LLC

Visit the Author Website at:
www.DianeKidman.com

Table of Contents

Introduction

We all have bad hair days. But if you're reaching for hats, barrettes, and headbands more often than not, you're probably thinking it's time for some major changes. Take a peek in your bathroom cabinet. How many half empty bottles of shampoo are hiding in there? Dusty bottles of conditioner? Hairspray that promised all-day hold and a silky gloss, but never did deliver on their promises? It's alright, you don't have to admit to the numbers. Truth is, I know exactly where you're coming from because I've been there.

After my son was born, it was as if every strand of hair on my head was replaced by strange mystery fibers. I wasn't able to style it and work with it as I once had, and even though I was using what I thought were top shelf shampoos and hair products, the results were getting less and less suitable for public viewing. I'd buy a bottle, use it a month, shove it in the cupboard after my hair tired of it, then I'd start the process all over again. It didn't matter if I was using chemical laden products or the most plant based stuff I could afford. They all ended up as part of my under-the-sink hair care memorial.

I tried numerous natural lines of hair care products. Some pretended to be natural with pretty flowers and leafy green things on the bottle, but the contents weren't natural at all. Others were 100% plant — I could almost hear the exotic birds every time I poured out the contents. Yet my hair still went limp after even the best of the bunch, was full of static during the winter months, and always snarled up, even when I used fancy conditioners. What was I going to do?

In a last ditch effort (it was either that or start shaving my head a la Sinead O'Connor), I started trying out natural remedies and making my own stuff. During my investigations, I stumbled across talk of the no 'poo movement which was being discussed across several online forums. What? Throw out the shampoo altogether? This sounded nuts! Just nuts enough for me to want to try it. And try it I did. I also gave myself a crash course in how to color my hair naturally, style it with homemade herbal products, and in essence, turn my furry mess into 100% chemical free, manageable hair. (Whether all you want are a few reliable hair recipes or you're ready to go all out with a no 'poo regimen, you'll find all those things and more in this book.)

As I gave up shampoo and went au naturale, I blogged my progress at www.dkMommySpot.com. While there was a short adjustment period, I noticed positive changes within a few days. After a few weeks, I was totally convinced. Four years later I still haven't shampooed my hair with anything out of a bottle. I still haven't poured smelly hair color on it. I haven't purchased a single bottle of shampoo, conditioner, hairspray, gel, or mousse. Now I make my own stuff.

Have I washed it? Absolutely, and regularly! My hair is shining. Clean, soft, not a snarl in it. I don't use a comb on my wet hair. Don't need to. I use my fingers because there are no knots or tangles, not ever, not even when I have longer hair. I haven't had a split end since 2008. I haven't had winter static, either.

I still have to style my hair, I still have "bad hair days," but it isn't due to a lack of volume or control. I'm a mom, which means most days I don't have the time to style it, much less look at myself in a mirror. But at least on those days it still feels great. It's healthy, clean, shining. And totally chemical free.

What's in the Book

In *Hair Gone Wild*, you'll get remedies to deal with all hair types and all hair conditions. Whether you've got fine blonde hair, coarse red hair, African or ethnic hair, curly, pin straight, or wavy, you'll find recipes and remedies you can use to improve the condition and gain control. You'll learn how to make your own hair care products like hairspray and gel, how to get rid of dandruff, how to make your hair stronger or more manageable, or how to combat hair loss. And you'll learn about the no 'poo process, which isn't as weird or as scary as it sounds.

What Exactly is No 'Poo?

It simply means choosing natural alternatives to the commercial synthetic products that so often contain harmful chemicals, including ingredients that straighten the hair, weigh it down, and strip it of sebum, which your hair needs to stay healthy. This means you use just a few common (and inexpensive) household items to clean your hair. Or herbal teas and essential oils to cleanse. If you still enjoy purchasing fancy bottles with high price tags, there are some mighty fine hair products available that are considered "no 'poo" but still look and feel like shampoo; however, our focus here will mainly be the do-it-yourself, herbal, simple ingredient approach.

Shampoo - A Brief History

If you'd like to envision a humankind without commercial shampoo, you won't have to travel back in time very far. In fact, let's hop back to 1914 when shampoo powder was first invented. If you were wealthy, you might get yourself some. You see, you'd need to be able to afford a hair stylist or a maid to wash your hair with the powder for you. It took time, several rinses, much scrubbing, and then styling afterwards, since your hair would be unmanageable after the whole ordeal. If you weren't wealthy, you might use a bar of soap every couple of months. Sure, come Saturday night you'd probably scrub your head in the bathtub, but soap was optional on the hair. In fact, one magazine article of the times that I read encouraged women to consider washing their hair as often as every four to six weeks.

I know what you're thinking here. Probably a great big "Ew," right? But let's think back to the old photographs we've seen of women's fashion at the turn of the 20th century. Keep in mind no stylish woman of the day would dare go out the day her hair was freshly washed, let alone get her photograph taken. She couldn't control her hair after a washing. So what you're seeing are photographs of no 'poo hair.

By the 1930s, the first commercial synthetic ingredient shampoo called Drene hit the market. While it quickly became one of the most heavily advertised items of the era, people still washed their hair much less frequently than we do now. In fact, one Drene advertisement I found stated that women should wash their hair the "Drene Way, which simply calls for one shampoo a week," four times more frequently than ever before.

So when did washing the hair become viewed as a daily necessity? Not until the 1970's when Farrah Fawcett showed us how lustrous our hair would flow if running down the beach in a bathing suit. Yes, we, too could have the glamorous locks of a super model if we used her Faberge shampoo. Every single day. For the first time, ever.

Before You Pitch the Shampoo

There are a few things to consider before letting the shampoo fly. Even if you're already certain you want to go no 'poo, you'll want to ask yourself a few questions in preparation. The last thing I want to do is to talk you out of the idea, but I also don't want you to give up after just a few days, as so many people do, because you weren't prepared for the transition. So let's take a look at a few common questions that many people have about the process.

How Soon Before My Hair Looks Great?

Yes, let's start with the important factor here. Leaving the shampoo aside means your hair will have a transition period. The good news is it doesn't last forever. The bad news? It exists. Your scalp contains sebaceous glands which produce an oil called sebum. That oil is good for your hair and is meant to protect it. Shampoo strips the hair of sebum, which causes the glands to kick out more of it, which causes you to shampoo more, which causes the glands to... Well, you get the point. In essence, the more you've shampooed, the more your hair wants to produce oil to protect against the damaging process.

When you first give up shampoo, it may seem as if your scalp is going haywire. It will produce more sebum, but hang tight — that's very temporary. Later on we'll discuss some ideas on how to get through that period as gracefully as possible. But the bottom line is, it usually takes less than a week for your hair to slow down sebum production, perhaps two to three weeks to totally kick the shampoo habit. Remember, while using shampoo, your hair probably feels oily before the end of the day. After your adjustment period is over, it'll take a few days, not a few hours, for your hair to feel oily between washes! And it'll look like a new head of hair.

What Will Other People Think?

We can say we don't care what others think, but there it is, we often do. Your decision to tell or not to tell is entirely up to you. If you are the type who enjoys a bit of confrontation, even verbal sparring, start telling all friends and family the day you give it up. Opinions vary, but for those who really adore shampoo, there's a good chance they'll be more than happy to tell you that you're crazy. Even after you've been at it for awhile and the results are great, there will always be someone who wants to act like there's something wrong with you because you don't fall for the shampoo thing anymore. Let them. Not everyone is as open minded as you!

I already mentioned that I announced my decision on my blog. That means I told thousands of people in one shot. But we're talking about like-minded people, and if I do say so, my readers are a supportive bunch who aren't afraid of trying something if it's natural, healthy, and produces better than average results.

I don't tell people I know personally unless they ask about my hair. My friends and family know I'm an all natural type, and on several occasions a friend or acquaintance has asked me what shampoo I use, expecting me to reveal a natural herbal wonder. I love watching their faces when I tell them I haven't shampooed in several years. The real testament is when they want all the details so they can consider trying it for themselves. Every one of those people have touched my hair like they can't believe it. I love that.

So whether or not you tell anyone is your business. But when they start asking you why your hair is so shiny or how come it's so curly all of a sudden, you're going to want to tell.

What Will My Hair Be Like the First Week?

Different. It's going to look and act different right away. The first couple of days may be an all-out revolt, so don't start your new regimen when you know you have a big meeting in two days. My advice? Take Friday as your first day to give up shampoo. Or some vacation time. Remember, I'll give you some hints on controlling your hair during this period.

The good news is, you'll see positive results almost immediately, and any weirdness is usually gone within a week. When I first went no 'poo, I took things quite literally and gave up everything, opting to wash with only water and an occasional vinegar or rosemary tea rinse. That lasted a couple of weeks before I decided I'd better find out how other people did it successfully. Nevertheless, I was amazed at how my hair — usually big unruly waves — was transforming into spiral curls. My hair also stood away from the scalp with body instead of laying flat against my head. Once I got on a good regimen, that's when things really took off and I began to figure out my hair's personality.

On the negative side, it may feel strange at first. That's okay, and you shouldn't let it scare you if you go through a short awkward stage. That's not what no 'poo hair feels like. It's just what your hair feels like for now. This too shall pass — and quickly.

Will No 'Poo Save Me Time?

It will take you a little less time to wash your hair the no 'poo way than it does with shampoo. There's no rinse and repeat. You still scrub and rinse, and you still condition if you so choose. (I'll share some good ones later — stuff you likely have already, and some really beautiful blends you can make yourself.) But it's easy enough that you'll have time to exfoliate, sing an aria, or perhaps knit something if you're into felting.

How to Wash Your Hair Without Shampoo

Now for the exciting part! You probably want to know what strange and exotic ingredients you'll need to hunt down to get going. You'll have to pack up and travel to the far reaches of your kitchen for the Big Three. What are the Big Three? Baking soda, apple cider vinegar, and honey. The honey is even optional, but if you've got coarse or dry hair, it'll become your favorite conditioner in a hurry.

Let's take a look at our ingredients, starting with the baking soda. I've often been asked where one can go to find aluminum-free baking soda. Actually, it's all aluminum free. The thing that sometimes contains aluminum is baking powder. Mixing the two items up is pretty common, so don't feel bad. I've done it myself, and while that batch of muffins was inedible, they did work fine for a family discus throwing event.

I'd love to recommend organic apple cider vinegar if you can get it. It may be a bit more expensive, but you'll need very little of it to keep you going. Compare that to a bottle of shampoo or conditioner, and you won't even flinch at the extra dollar or two.

Lastly, let's talk honey. I'm not very particular about a brand or whether it's clover, wildflower, deep woods pine, etc. Just honey. In a cute bottle, preferably a bear. (You'll be keeping it in the shower, so he'll make you smile on a Monday morning.)

It's also good to have a couple containers at the ready. I use a metal water bottle and an unbreakable mug.

Before showering, put one tablespoon of baking soda in a container such as a water bottle, and add 12 to 16 ounces of water. (Hot water makes for a more comfortable wash, but cold water makes the hair smoother and softer.) Cap and shake so all the baking soda is dissolved.

In a mug or cup, put one or two tablespoons of apple cider vinegar. Put both the baking soda water and the cup with vinegar at arm's reach near the shower.

In the shower, thoroughly wet down your hair. Next, slowly pour the baking soda water over your hair. You need not use the whole bottle. Just pour enough over your hair to saturate it with the mixture. That is usually somewhere between ⅓ and ½ the bottle. Now massage it into your hair, paying most of your attention to scrubbing your scalp, in particular the crown of your head which tends to produce more oils. There's really no need to worry about scrubbing at your hair, believe it or not. Taking care to cleanse your scalp is the key. The baking soda will take care of your hair for you.

Leave the baking soda water on your head for a minute or two. Now rinse your hair thoroughly, again concentrating on massaging the scalp.

Take the mug or cup containing one or two tablespoons of vinegar and fill it the rest of the way with warm water from your shower. Slowly pour it over your head, saturating all your hair. Massage it into your scalp well, then rinse it out thoroughly.

That's all there is to it! The whole process will take you less time than the explanation just did.

In the beginning, you might feel like using the baking soda wash and vinegar rinse every day, but every other day (every third for some people, even once a week) will work very well. On alternate days, I like to use honey as a conditioning treatment, and I've noticed it does have a cleaning effect too, albeit a lighter one. If you use the baking soda and cider vinegar daily, it's easy to end up with hair that's too dry. So don't overdo it.

To condition with honey, pour about a teaspoon to a tablespoon of honey into the palm of your hand and use it just like you would any conditioner. Massage it in, let it sit for a few seconds or a minute, then rinse it out. While you may be envisioning a sticky mess and an unpleasant sensation putting honey on your hair, it isn't at all. Since it's water soluble, it works into the hair and rinses back out easily.

You'll quickly learn new things about your hair that perhaps you never knew before. Maybe you'll find out you have curly hair when you thought it was just unmanageable waves. Or perhaps after a few weeks, you'll discover that your hair likes it best when you do the baking soda wash and the cider rinse a mere two times a week.

Adjusting the ratios is easy if you keep an eye out for a few things. If, for instance, your hair starts to seem too dry to you, use a bit more cider in your cider rinse and/or less baking soda rinse. Too oily or flat? Try less cider. (I used to use ½ cup cider to ½ cup water! I found I was overdoing it by quite a large margin. It's much happier with less, and yours will be too.)

During winter months, keeping the honey on your hair longer can help combat dryness, while summertime weather may require using honey only once a week. It's all a matter of tweaking, which beats having to change shampoos every time your hair wants to play "hide the volume" on you.

Getting Through the Transition Process with Ease

For some, the changes are immediate and drastic. There's no looking back from the first wash, and if that's you, congratulations! You just got over your shampoo addiction easily. But for others, dumping the suds means feeling about as awkward as a high school girl with a pimple on prom night. How do you get through it without giving up?

First, make sure to concentrate on any small improvements in your hair. Most people are immediately impressed with the changes, so focus on those as best you can. Remember, it's all a matter of time. Once you get over the hump, it's all downhill.

The one thing you do not want to do — under any circumstances — is to use shampoo "just once," thinking you'll go back to more natural means the following day. I can tell you from experience that's the worst thing you can do.

After a few weeks of going without shampoo, I thought I'd go for a haircut. Very bad idea. (Get the haircut *before* giving up shampoo so you're completely over the transition period before the next cut is needed!) I washed my hair and went into the stylist's still wet. I was too embarrassed to tell her I was no 'poo. Yes, I know. I should have told her. But I didn't.

I did, however, tell her that I'd just washed and there was no need for her to do so. Since my hair was barely damp by that point, she said she'd just wet it down. But in our torrent of conversation, she grabbed the shampoo bottle anyway. Although when she realized what she'd done, she didn't bother to scrub it in but rinsed it out right away instead, the deed was done. I went home, blow dried, and just about cried when I saw the limp, flat, disgusting mess upon my head. The professional salon shampoo that was once upon a time my favorite brand had sabotaged my hair. I looked like a drowned rat and remained in that state for well over a week, losing large handfuls of hair every day in the shower. I'm not exactly sure why I was losing so much hair, but my guess is that I was no longer used to the chemicals and ingredients in shampoo. My hair revolted against the attack and let me know by dropping dead. That was back in 2008, the last time my hair saw shampoo.

Moral of the story? Don't cheat.

So what do you do to get through a rough patch? You could try a rosemary tea rinse, which helps control excess oil, gets rid of dandruff, increases hair growth, decreases hair loss, and gives a fantastic shine. You can use a rosemary tea any day you wish; whether it's a washing day or an in-between day.

Purchase dried rosemary in bulk from a health food store or online. It's very inexpensive. Prepare a strong tea the night before (or at least an hour before) by pouring boiling water over a teaspoon of rosemary in a tea ball. Let it steep anywhere from one hour to overnight, then strain. Pour it over wet hair. No need to rinse it back out. Just massage it in, then style as usual. Your hair will look shiny and smell wonderful. (It's not a flowery smell, either, so it's not just for the girls.)

If you use rosemary on a regular basis, it may darken your hair a bit. Blondes might consider using a chamomile rinse, redheads a calendula rinse; same as described above. All three offer up shine and a fresh, clean smell. (More herbal teas that make great color rinses will be discussed later.)

Remember, don't allow yourself to get frustrated. Sure, a ponytail or a hat may be in order at first, but those days will be few if you keep at it. Keep a journal, mark your calendar for the day you gave it all up, brag about it when people start asking why your hair looks so full and healthy.

Hair Remedies for All Kinds of Things

Essential Oils and Herbal Teas for Hair Health

If you've given up the shampoo, you'll need to know what you can rely on to keep your hair shining and healthy, no matter your newfound hair type. Essential oils and dried herbs offer up solutions to all sorts of hair issues and can be used in a myriad of ways. We'll discuss those ways, but first let's look at essential oils and dried herbs by hair type. Once you've identified if your hair is normal or oily, dry or in need of treatment for dandruff — perhaps a bit of each — you can choose a combination of oils and dried herbs depending on your experiences, your fragrance preference, your mood.

Essential Oils by Hair Type

Dry: Chamomile, lavender, palmarosa, rose geranium, rosemary, rosewood, sandalwood, wintergreen

Oily: Clary sage, cedarwood, cypress, lemon, lemongrass, patchouli, petitgrain, sage

All Hair Types: Carrot seed, lavender, Roman chamomile, rosemary

Dandruff: Basil, cedarwood, cypress, geranium, juniper, lavender, rosemary, sage, spearmint, tea tree, thyme, wintergreen

Hair Loss & Balding: Cedarwood, clary sage, cypress, lavender, lemon, peppermint, Roman chamomile, rosemary, rose geranium, sage, sage lavender, spikenard, thyme, wintergreen, ylang-ylang

Growth Stimulation: Basil, cedarwood, cypress, ginger, grapefruit, hyssop, lavender, lemon, rose geranium, rosemary, sage, thyme, ylang ylang

Dried Herbs by Hair Type

Dry: Calendula, chamomile, comfrey, lavender, orange peel (organic), rosemary, sandalwood, burdock root

Oily: Burdock, lemongrass, lemon peel (organic), sage

All Hair Types: Chamomile, lavender, rose, rosemary

Dandruff: Burdock, sage, willow bark

Hair Loss & Balding: Nettle, peppermint

Preparing Your Rinse

Once you've chosen a dried herb and an essential oil (or combination of each) that you'd like to try, you'll need to prepare the rinse. This is easy, and the mixes can be stored in the refrigerator for up to three days before it's time to make a fresh batch. You may choose to use your rinse every day, once a week, or at a whim.

Prepare one pint of the herbal tea of your choice by pouring nearly boiling water over the herbs. (Remember, loose leaf tea is always cheaper. Get a tea ball so you don't have to mess with straining the herb.) Cover and allow the tea to steep for at least 30 minutes. Strain, then add just 3 drops of essential oils and 1 tablespoon apple cider vinegar. Pour on your head and allow it to sit for a few minutes before rinsing out. This is a nice amped up alternative to the apple cider rinse you'd usually use after washing with baking soda water.

You can also use a little essential oil directly on your hair if you're cautious. One drop of lavender or rosemary oil is nice for any hair type; sandalwood is especially nice on dry, split ends. Rub the oil in the palms of your hands and massage it into the ends of your hair. Don't put essential oil directly onto your scalp, however. And don't use more than a drop. Essential oil can get drying if used in larger amounts, and you can develop an allergy to the herbs if you get too enthusiastic with your usage.

Natural Dandruff Treatments

Some people experience a kicking up of the dandruff when they first give up shampoo. If you're sure it's dandruff and not just an overdose of too much baking soda which can cause a buildup if you're too heavy handed with it, then you're no doubt anxious to end the problem. While this is often just a temporary side effect during the no 'poo transition stage, here are several more remedies to tackle an itchy, flaky scalp, and to allow you to once more enjoy that black turtleneck collection of yours.

Scalp Oil Dandruff Treatment

Massage oils are a good way to treat the scalp. Mix 25 drops of the dandruff-fighting essential oil of your choice with 2 ounces of aloe juice (not gel) or jojoba oil, massage your scalp with the mixture, and leave it on for a couple of hours before washing it out. This treatment can be done daily as needed.

Burdock & Herbs Dandruff Snuffer

The following recipe is very effective. While one version I found requires a cup of fresh peach tree leaves, you can make it with or without. My version is without since that'd mean you can only prepare this treatment either in warm weather only, or if you live somewhere in Georgia. Also, fruit trees are often heavily sprayed. But if you've got your very own untreated peach tree and it's June, why not throw in the peach leaves too?

What You'll Need:

1 cup dried burdock root (chopped or powdered)
1 cup dried chamomile
½ cup dried sage leaves
8 cups apple cider vinegar
A large glass jar with a tight fitting lid

Put all the ingredients into the glass jar and allow it to steep for two weeks. In a warm, not hot, location is best. Herbs like sunny windows. I think they feel good there. Strain out the herbs and pour some of the herb vinegar into a spray bottle. Saturate your scalp every evening and don't rinse it out until morning. This serves as your shampoo as well. Just rinsing out your hair and scrubbing the scalp is enough to have clean, dandruff-free hair.

A vinegar like this has a good long shelf life if stored in a cool, dark location after the herb has been strained out. You should be able to hang onto it for several years. If it starts to look or smell different, it's time to dump it out and make a fresh batch.

If you'd like to darken your hair while fighting the dandruff, you can even add a cup of dried hops to the other herbs for steeping.

The Parsley Trick

Easier than the previous method with a lot less preparation, a nice parsley tea will help stomp out dandruff. Using just ½ cup chopped parsley (curly or flat, this isn't a fussy cooking show), pour 2 cups boiling water over the herb and let it sit for 30 minutes before use. After washing your hair, massage it into the scalp and allow it to stay on for several minutes before rinsing out. Or keep it in. Don't worry. You won't smell like a garnish.

Nettle Vinegar

Stinging nettle (*Urtica dioica*) is so much more than a weed that bites you when you garden. It's probably just trying to get your attention because it knows how fabulous it is. Loaded with vitamins and minerals, we should all be drinking the tea. Which makes me think. I need to stop everything and get me a stinging nettle tea. But before I run off to brew, let me tell you how to prepare this vinegar rinse for dandruff.

Steep 4 tablespoons of dried stinging nettle in 2 cups of almost boiling water. Let it sit a good 30 minutes before straining it out. Once it's cool, mix it with a cup of apple cider vinegar and store it all in a clean glass container. Massage it into your scalp whenever you need it. You can do this before washing if you allow it to dry first, before bed, or whenever the itch hits.

Now, if you'll excuse me, I have a nettle tea to prepare. Without the vinegar. I plan to drink it.

Anti-Dandruff Ginger Rinse

This rinse uses fresh ginger as a dander combatant. It's also a nice way to encourage blood circulation to the scalp.

1 oz. fresh ginger, minced
1 oz. dried chamomile flowers
1 gallon purified water
cheesecloth

Put the ginger and chamomile in the cheesecloth and tie it shut with string. Place it in a pot with the water, and boil for ten minutes. Allow it to cool, then remove the cheesecloth. After washing your hair, massage ½ to 1 ounce of the rinse into your scalp. Don't rinse this back out. You can store the rest of the rinse in the refrigerator for later use. This usually keeps about three days.

Aloe Vera Dandruff Kicker-Outer

Aloe on its own has a way of scaring away dandruff and any other scalp issues you may have. As always, make sure the aloe gel you have is pure stuff. I've seen some scary products in the stores going undercover as aloe gel. Here's a hint: If it glows greener than Kryptonite, it's not natural. If it smells like ocean breezes at a tropical resort, it's not natural. And if the ingredients listed say anything but "aloe vera gel," it's not natural. Your best bet is to invest in a nice big potted aloe vera plant. You don't even need to water it very often; it prefers neglect, which is probably why mine thrives so.

To use aloe for dandruff or any other scalp issue, massage the gel into the scalp at night. In the morning when you wet down your hair in the shower, scrub your scalp just like you would for washing. The aloe on your head will even offer a bit of foaming action. No need to use any cleansers on your hair other than this when you do the aloe treatment.

Scalp Itch Eraser

If your scalp is itchy and tight but dandruff isn't necessarily the problem, you could use a bit of scalp conditioning. I found this old-time remedy in a turn-of-the-century beauty book, and the ingredients are definitely scalp friendly and itch reducing.

Apply the whites of two eggs to your scalp by using your fingers to rub it in. Rinse the egg whites out with the juice of two lemons that have been diluted in a quart of cool water.

Keep in mind lemon juice has the ability to lighten hair if you go in the sun afterwards.

Hair Loss, Balding, and Promoting Hair Growth

If you've decided to give up shampoo, you're already well on your way to restoring your hair's health. You'll probably find less hair in the tub, in the brush, and on the floor. After a few months, you may notice new hair growth — stubby little hairs at the temples, along the hairline, making their way into the world and filling in those voids on your scalp. But if you're not seeing enough of a change, all is not lost. What follows is a wide variety of treatments, from hair oils and lotions to herbs and dietary changes.

Massage Oil for the Balding & Thinning Scalp

If you've got any hair loss concerns at all, the first and foremost treatment you should concern yourself with is massaging the scalp. Even if you have no hair loss issues but want healthier, fuller hair, massaging is key. It promotes hair growth — faster hair growth — like nothing else. Hair can't grow without sufficient blood circulation in the scalp.

Massaging is the best way to accomplish that. Don't be too vigorous. The point here is to stimulate, not to scrape and scratch. Just use your fingertips to work in a gentle circular motion. You can do this anytime, anywhere, except when you're driving or in heavy combat situations.

To aid in your scalp massage, you can add some homemade herbal massage oil, which will give the hair growth a boost. The following recipe contains rosemary, which is a fine essential oil for hair. A rubefacient, it promotes blood circulation, thus giving hair a nice place to grow. (Rosemary oil will not darken the hair like the tea, so it's fine for any hair color and type.)

What You'll Need:

50 drops rosemary essential oil
½ cup natural aloe vera gel (That means nothing with additives. Just pure gel.)
1 Tbs. apple cider vinegar
1 Tbs. jojoba oil

Pour contents into a bottle and cap it. Shake well before each use. Every evening, massage a small amount into your scalp, taking your time to work it in. A good ten minutes of massage would be perfect. If you're concerned about ruining bedding, you can place an old towel on your pillowcase. In the morning, wash it out.

The "Baldness is the Pits" Remedy

We talked about peach leaves a bit earlier, but there's another part of the peach that likes to help out when the hair isn't staying on top of things. Peach seeds, which reside like a nut inside the pit, would like to offer their own remedy. No need to go out and purchase a peck of peaches. You can buy peach seeds at many health food stores in bulk and online. Make sure they're not old, though. And if you've got organic? All the better!

Boil ½ cup of the peach seeds in 2 cups of apple cider vinegar until the vinegar gets nice and thick. Wait for it to cool, then store it in a glass container with a tight lid. Massage it into your scalp well, and allow it to sit for a few minutes before washing it back out. You can store this in the fridge for later use. The vinegar works as a natural preservative, but keep an eye on it to make sure the look and smell of it doesn't alter. If it does, time to prepare some fresh.

Scalp Conditioner

This oil blend features olive oil, a fine hair remedy indeed. It offers a deep conditioning for the hair while the essential oils go to work on hair growth. This would double nicely as a dandruff control oil.

What You'll Need:

1 tsp. rosemary essential oil
5 drops lemongrass essential oil
½ cup olive oil (The better the quality, the better the results. Always use fresh, not rancid smelling.)

Blend the oils together in a clean jar and cap tightly. Shake to mix. In the evening, massage it into your scalp for ten minutes. Sleep with an old towel on your pillow to avoid staining bedding. In the morning, wash it out thoroughly.

Minty Rinse

Prepare a cup of peppermint tea, allowing it to steep for at least 15 minutes. Add a tablespoon of vinegar and use this as your final rinse in the shower. You can rinse it out or leave it. The vinegar smell will dissipate in short order.

Gingko Biloba

Gingko biloba not only improves memory and brain function, it improves circulation to the scalp as well. Try 40 to 60 mg of gingko (tablet form) two to three times daily for an internal boost. (Maybe you'll stop losing those car keys, too.)

Other Considerations

There are numerous reasons for hair loss. We all lose some — about 50 to 70 strands of head hair a day — but when it doesn't grow back, that's when the concern begins. Sometimes hair loss is prompted by long term illness, getting off of oral contraceptives, giving birth, miscarriage, abortion, or going through a life changing or traumatic experience. Don't forget to look at things like diet, lifestyle, and medications.

I have a strange hobby: I read warnings on popular prescriptions. Perhaps "hobby" is a strong word choice here, but when I offer to help someone with a health issue, I like to start with a good look at their medications. You'd be amazed at how many popular prescription meds cause hair loss, not to mention things much worse. If a prescription you're taking has hair loss as a possible side effect, all the massaging in the world might do nothing. So talk to your doctor about alternatives.

Stress is a pretty big trigger for hair loss. Ever had a cat? Nothing makes a cat shed faster than adding a Doberman to the room or going to Thailand for a month without letting her know first. Good news is, take the Doberman out of the room and Fluffy stops throwing fur all over the place. If you're losing hair, my advice is to take the Doberman out of the room.

When looking over your diet, be sure to take an honest look at how much processed food and refined sugar you consume each day. Fatty foods? Not good. Essential fatty acids found in things like beans and avocados? Good. On the other end of the spectrum, if you're a chronic dieter who avoids fats altogether, you could be starving your hair. Balance is key.

If your hair loss is sudden and you can't trace it to things like stress, diet, or medications, take a visit to your doctor.

Deep Conditioning Treatments

Just because you've gone no 'poo doesn't mean your hair will behave itself immediately. By the time your hair reaches your shoulders, it's about 3 years old. That means that depending on how long your hair is, you'll be hanging out with chemically treated and commercially shampooed hair for awhile.

For me, that meant I had to grow out color treated hair. I had been using an (almost) natural version of a boxed hair color which worked well and didn't smell so bad, but I didn't want to do anything harsh to my hair anymore. What I wanted to do was to try and restore my previously tortured tresses until all the damage grew out and was cut off. That's where deep conditioning comes in.

Holy Guacamole Deep Conditioning

Let's start with a simple one: avocado. It's full of essential fatty acids, and if you eat these on a regular basis, you can help your hair and skin from the inside out. But as a deep conditioner, you can apply avocado directly to your hair. Just smash the avocado like you would to make a guacamole. Smear the avocado on clean hair (damp or dry), then wait five minutes before rinsing it out thoroughly. Do it once a week or as needed. (I'll bring the chips.)

Coconut Oil Conditioning

For a visit to the tropics, grab some good organic virgin coconut oil. It's a longtime favorite for deep conditioning treatments or a light leave-in and a popular choice in India where the women are known for their healthy hair. Scientific studies have shown that the hair shaft absorbs it well unlike other oils, and that it reduces protein loss in both damaged and undamaged hair.

Coconut oil looks like a solid until it's exposed to low heat. Just rubbing some between your palms is enough to liquefy it for use. To use as a deep conditioner, apply it to your hair in the evening and either use a shower cap or cover your pillow with an old towel to protect bedding. Wash it out in the morning.

I often use coconut oil at night before bed, but in a small quantity. I work it into my hair, especially the ends. I don't use much (maybe the size of a small pea), and I do it perhaps a half hour before bed allowing my hair a chance to soak it up. It absorbs surprisingly well and has made a remarkable improvement in my hair's quality.

As a leave-in conditioner, apply a very small amount to the ends and dry areas after washing and drying. I also love coconut oil as a light moisturizer, especially for sunny summertime skin.

Mineral Hair Mask

For this do-it-yourself mineral hair mask, you'll probably have to stop at the health food store first or do a bit of online shopping. The minerals in our recipe are found in bentonite clay, which has the ability to remove heavy metals. It can remove residues from the scalp, along with any fungal issues responsible for itching. It's a good masque for all hair types, in particular African hair.

What You'll Need:

¼ cup bentonite clay
¼ cup rosemary tea (brewed strong)
½ cup sage tea (brewed strong)

Prepare a paste of the clay and teas so you have a nice consistency that will allow for easy application without dripping. Apply the masque to just damp hair with a spatula or with your hands, being sure to cover the whole head. Cover your hair with a plastic bag, plastic wrap, or a shower cap, then wrap your head in a nice warm towel. Allow the masque to sit for 15 to 20 minutes before thoroughly rinsing with cool water.

Protein Conditioner

Protein. It makes you strong, it makes your hair strong too. Try this conditioner to give your hair a boost of health.

1 egg white
5 Tbs. yogurt (plain; not fat free)

Beat the egg white until it's foamy, then add the yogurt and mix it well. Apply the mixture to your hair, small areas at a time to ensure you cover it all. Leave it in for 15 minutes before rinsing.

Conditioning Honey Prewash

Treat your hair occasionally to this soft and luxurious conditioning treatment. You can use it before you wash your hair, or it can replace that day's washing. Either way, the results are clean and smooth.

½ cup honey
3 tsp. warm olive oil (not hot!)
4 drops rosemary essential oil

Mix the ingredients together well, then apply it all over damp hair. A squeeze bottle works well here. Massage it into your scalp making sure all hair is coated. Cover your hair with a warm towel or a shower cap. Leave it in for 30 minutes before rinsing it out with cool water.

Herbal Hair Oil for Dry, Damaged Hair

If you've put your hair through the ringer in the past with all manner of frying and drying, a good hair oil will be your new best friend. This one infuses several herbs known for their healing properties. Apply a very small amount to your hair by rubbing it in your palms and working it into the damaged areas, especially the ends. Alternatively, you can mix some of the hair oil in a 50/50 mixture with honey and saturate your hair with it, then cover your hair with a warm towel. Wait 30 minutes before washing it out.

What You'll Need:

1 part dried burdock
1 part dried marshmallow
1 part dried nettle
1 part dried parsley

Crush the herbs slightly with a mortar and pestle and place them in a clean, dry jar. Fill the jar with olive oil until the herbs are covered completely. You can push the herbs down with a wooden chopstick, working as many air bubbles out as

you can before capping tightly. Allow the mixture to steep for
two weeks before straining.

Hair Oil with Rosemary

Here's another simple hair oil. Again, apply just a few drops
of the oil to your palms, then rub the palms together before
working the oil into the ends of the hair.

3 oz. sweet almond oil
30 drops cinnamon essential oil
30 drops rosemary essential oil

Blend the three oils together in a bottle, and store in a cool
dark place.

Banana Cream Conditioner

Guaranteed to make you hungry, this conditioner is dessert for
your hair. Use this one before you wash your hair.

1 smashed banana

2 - 3 tsp. olive oil

4 - 5 tsp. milk (avoiding the fat free variety is best but not necessary)

Mix ingredients well and apply to freshly brushed or combed hair. Allow it to sit for 15 to 20 minutes before rinsing with lukewarm water. Wash your hair to remove any remaining oil. Steer clear of monkeys.

Cocoa Hair Butter

Hair butters are a great way to bring moisture to the hair. They're slightly solid in nature, much like a salve, and can be used as often as you like. This first version relies on fragrant cocoa butter to humectify dry hair.

What You'll Need:

1 oz. sweet almond oil
2 oz. jojoba oil
8 oz. cocoa butter
A few drops essential oil of choice

Fill a saucepan halfway with water. Place the cocoa butter, sweet almond oil, and jojoba in a heatproof measuring cup, and put the cup in the saucepan. Slowly heat the cocoa butter until it's all melted, then remove from heat. Add essential oils if using, then pour the mixture into a clean dry jar. Wait for the hair butter to cool fully before capping tightly. To use, melt a very small amount between the palms of your hands, rubbing your hands together until it's liquefied. Work the hair butter into the ends of your hair to prevent split ends and soften the hair.

Shea Hair Butter

Here's another version of hair butter, this time with shea butter being the magic ingredient.

What You'll Need:

1 oz. jojoba oil
½ oz. sweet almond oil
8 oz. shea butter
A few drops essential oil of your choice

Put the jojoba oil, sweet almond oil, and shea butter into a glass heatproof measuring cup. Fill a saucepan halfway with water, and place the measuring cup inside the saucepan. Slowly heat the oils until the shea butter is completely dissolved. Remove from the heat and add essential oils if using. Pour mixture into a clean dry glass jar, and wait for the hair butter to completely cool before capping tightly. Melt a small amount of the butter between your palms by rubbing your hands together until it's liquefied. Work the butter into the ends of your hair for split end prevention and the softening of the hair.

Lentil Orange Water for Oily Hair

If after giving up shampoo your hair still insists on being on the oily side, try this unique oily hair remedy. Soak one lentil of any variety in a glass of water for 30 minutes, then remove the lentil. Peel an orange (organic) and boil the rind in water. Mix the orange water with the lentil water and use as your final rinse. Alternatively, put two or three drops of sweet orange oil in the water and stir well with a chopstick or stirring tool designated just for your essential oil experiments.

Orris Root Dry Shampoo (Old-Fashioned Airing Powder)

Old-fashioned dry shampoo blends show up occasionally in old formularies and remedy books. This one is wonderfully fragrant, faintly reminiscent of violets thanks to the orris root, and absorbs excess oils in the hair. If you have long hair and don't like to bother with wetting and drying all the time, you can opt to use this powder instead of a dowse in the shower.

What You'll Need:

2 quart glass jar (A canning jar is perfect.)
3 ½ cups orris root powder
3 cups cornstarch
5 drops rosemary essential oil
5 drops lavender essential oil
2 or 3 dried rosebuds or rose petals (Organic or dried especially for tea is best; dried from the florist may contain lots of pesticides.)

Put the orris root and cornstarch in the jar, then close the jar and roll it. Don't shake it or you'll have a fog of a mess when you need to open it back up. Wait a few minutes for the dust to settle, then put the essential oils on the rosebuds or petals. Place the roses in the jar with the powder and roll it again. If it's spring and you have access to fresh violet flowers, you can add several handfuls to the mix as well. Put the jar in a dark place and wait three weeks, rolling it occasionally to aid in blending.

To use the powder, put one or two tablespoons in a salt shaker, preferably one with tiny holes. This is a fine powder! Part your hair and put a very light sprinkling at the scalp. Continue parting your hair and sprinkling, gently working in the powder with your fingers. Using a clean brush, brush the powder through the hair to the ends. You can then take a square of cheesecloth (just one layer is fine) and push it over your brush. Work back through your hair with the brush to remove powder.

Chlorine Eliminator Mask

For swimmers, getting the chlorine out of your hair is a difficult task without the aid of chemically shampoos. But the following recipe gives you the natural remedy your hair was hoping for.

What You'll Need:

1 beaten egg

2 Tbs. olive oil

¼ c. pureed peeled cucumber

Combine the ingredients, then massage into your hair from the scalp to the tips. Cover your head with a shower cap and steep yourself for 30 minutes to an hour, keeping your hair at room temperature. Don't heat your hair, or you'll ruin the effect, not to mention frying the egg. Wash mixture from hair. Repeat as necessary.

Coloring Your Hair with Henna & Friends

Now that your hair is 100% chemical free and feeling more balanced, you'll want to keep it that way. If you're used to coloring your hair, that means finding alternatives. The good news is, there are some very impressive hair coloring herbs that can be tweaked to deliver just the color you want. I've been using henna for years, and I love it. It's permanent, covers the gray (not that I have any. Ahem!) and it eliminates dandruff, thickens the hair, and adds great shine. Not the redhead type? No problem! You can add other herbs to henna to alter the shades, or go with a different herb altogether for variations on color. There are even easy color rinses for temporary color that we'll cover after the more permanent options.

It's important to note that the end result of henna — or any of the following herbs — depends largely on the color of your hair to begin with. Henna adds red to whatever you have right now. Blonde hair will become bright (but not brassy) red, gray hair will be a bright strawberry blonde, brown hair will become auburn, and African hair will be black with deep red highlights. Henna works great on white hair as well, turning it a nice light auburn. If you normally have coarse and/or curly hair, it can soften it and relax it somewhat. (This doesn't seem to be the case for everyone, but it does have this effect on me.)

Important Note: This is just to give you a rough idea of color. The only way to find out what color your hair will become while using henna or ANY herb on your hair is to do a strand test first. You can remove hair from your brush if you don't want to cut a piece. Follow the instructions below for your desired hair color, test the strand, then wait a few days to see how the hair oxidizes. (Coloring your hair with herbs usually requires a few days before the true color fully emerges.) Also, you'll want to test a bit on your skin in an inconspicuous location to make sure you're not allergic to the herbs or the lemon juice. If you're too sensitive to lemon juice, you can use orange juice or grapefruit juice in place of lemon.

Purchasing your henna is an important step. Not all henna is created equal. For instance, I've seen it offered in little bottles in exotic food stores. But these bottles contain things other than just henna. We're going to mix our own because we want to know what we're getting. What you should look for is dried, powdered henna. Some companies will state their henna is for body art, and that's great — as long as it's body art quality henna and not a pre-made mix or a blend, and you shouldn't buy the stuff in a tube thinking it'll save time. Not the same.

How Much Henna?

For short hair, you'll need about 100 grams; shoulder length, 200 - 300 grams; longer hair needs 400 - 500 grams. Guess on the high side to be safe. Nice thing about henna? Once you've prepared it, you can freeze the leftovers for later use.

I purchase my henna from my neighborhood health food store. The brand they sell is from Frontier Co-op, which is also available online, and it's inexpensive and works very well. It always seems fresh and fragrant, and I can buy it in big one-pound bags. Wherever you choose to get your henna, make sure it has a nice green color and that it smells full and fresh.

There are plenty of places that sell henna at exorbitant prices claiming to be of extraordinary quality. While I can't vouch for everyone out there, I did once take a chance on an expensive box of henna. I couldn't tell the least bit of difference between it and what I was already using. So if money is a factor, don't feel like you have to take out a second mortgage to color your hair. Some of the lower priced brands do the trick nicely; just be sure to take the time to get the right stuff.

What you'll need:

powdered henna (amount determined by length as discussed earlier)
20 to 40 ounces lemon juice
glass or enamel bowl
spoon
plastic gloves
several feet of plastic wrap, folded and set nearby
old towel (at least one - two may be better)
garbage bag for refuse
cotton balls
2 - 4 hours to sit, relax, read a book, etc. (Not the day to paint the living room, for instance.)

Henna works best when it's prepared with lemon juice. To make the process easier on you, try to go with a bottled lemon juice that contains no preservatives or additives — it should be straight lemon. Squeezing lemons will work, but it does make the process more lengthy and not so enjoyable, not to mention a little seedy. Besides, you need a whole lot of lemons, usually at least a dozen. I buy bottles of organic lemon juice at Costco, and many health food stores carry all natural lemon juice too.

If lemon juice proves to be irritating for you, you can use ½ lemon juice with ½ distilled water, or use orange or grapefruit juice instead of lemon. But don't use only water; some people suggest boiling water, but that makes for a brassy color that fades.

Mix the henna in a bowl, preferably glass or enamel, the night before you intend to use it. Keep in mind henna is messy stuff and does stain things easily, so for mixing purposes, try putting the bowl in the kitchen sink. Carefully pour the powdered henna into the bowl. Add some lemon juice and stir the mixture. You'll want to continually add the juice little by little, working out the lumps. The end consistency should be something like thick frosting for a cake or mashed potatoes. You'll be thinning it out a bit in the morning.

If you can't get all the lumps out for now, that's okay. They have a way of disappearing after several hours. Cover the bowl and leave it in the sink overnight. Twelve hours is ideal. Warn the family not to mess with it, and that it is not dark green pudding left there for their enjoyment.

In the morning, give the henna a good stirring, and add a splash more lemon juice to it until it's about the consistency of a thick yogurt. Now you're ready to henna your hair.

Before you start, be sure to prepare your work area. If you're applying the henna by leaning over the side of the tub, for instance, be sure to remove bath mats and good towels, pull back the shower curtain — whatever you don't want to turn red. Place down old towels or some sort of protection if you have floors you're worried about. As for your bathtub, I've personally not had any issues with it staining an average fiberglass tub. But you don't want it getting on grout. Any slopped henna can usually be removed if you get to it right away with a damp cloth, perhaps with some lemon juice on it, so keep some rags nearby just in case. In essence, if you've ever colored your own hair at home, you already know what to move out of the way.

You'll need your hair to be clean and dry. I find it's easier to tell where you've already applied the henna if your hair is dry at the start, especially if you're relying on touch only and not a mirror.

Make sure you have a long piece of plastic wrap close enough that you can reach it easily. Pull on your gloves and part your hair. You're going to apply the henna with your fingers (or use a plastic bag and "pipe" it on like cake decorating), starting at the scalp first. Work your way down the part in your hair, applying as you go, making sure to get right up to the scalp. Manipulate the henna with your fingers for thorough application. Fully coat each section of hair like smoothing on mud. Part your hair again, an inch or less over from the first spot, and apply more henna. Work your way through your entire head, making sure to put plenty on. The more you thoroughly cover your hair, the better. Be sure to coat the hairline, including temples, forehead, behind ears, etc. It's helpful to have a hand mirror where you can get at it, just to make sure you didn't miss anything.

Once your head is covered fully, wrap the plastic wrap around and around your head like a big turban. Be as careful as you can to get as much of your hair covered as possible. Take an old damp rag or damp paper towels and wipe away any excess on the skin around the hair line, making sure to check around (and sometimes in) your ears. If it looks like it's staining you, you can remove it with a bit of lemon juice. If it's a faint stain, don't worry. That usually goes away the next time you wash your hair.

Cotton balls are optional, but you can tuck those into the plastic wrap around your hair line if you're worried about anything sneaking out. I also wrap an old towel around my shoulders and clip it into place.

This is the point where I rinse down the tub and check to make sure I didn't inadvertently slap a glob of henna somewhere unexpected, like on the tile or a wandering dog. Once that bit of house upkeep is done, it's off to read a book or settle in somewhere cozy for awhile. The henna should remain on your hair for two to four hours (four if you have dye-resistant hair), so grab an old movie, read a book outdoors where the sun can help warm the henna, or enjoy a snooze.

If you're anywhere as impatient as I am, all this waiting might sound just short of painful. But I assure you the results are worth it, and after using henna on my hair for several years, I never give the wait a second thought. I just wrap my head up and go about my business. And I don't answer the door anymore. (That last little kid will never forgive me.)

After your waiting is done, put your gloves back on. Then pull off the plastic wrap in one big piece. Toss it in the garbage bag you have ready, then start rinsing. Rinse very well until the water runs clear. I like to finish things up by massaging a few tablespoons of honey into my hair. I let it sit for a minute or two, then I rinse it back out. It gives a nice extra conditioning. I've heard lots of henna users say they feel no need for conditioning afterwards, but it's always worked best for me when I do.

Dry and style as usual. You'll notice that after a couple of days go by, the color seems to "settle." It will deepen slightly and become a bit richer as the henna oxidizes. You'll also notice your hair will be incredibly soft and shiny, and any dandruff you did have is magically gone.

To me, henna has an earthy smell that reminds me of fallen leaves and autumn. If you don't like the smell of henna, you can rinse your hair with rosemary tea or with water that has a drop or two of essential oil in it. The smell will fade over a few washings, but the color won't.

Using Henna and Indigo for Brown Shades

You can also get your hair various shades of brown by adding indigo to your henna treatment. (Later we'll discuss getting a dramatic black with indigo.) You have to use it with henna even if you're not interested in reds, because indigo on its own will leave you blue. Remember where your jeans get their color, after all!

Sometimes indigo is referred to as "black" henna, but it's best to get indigo that's not labeled as such so you don't accidentally get something that's not pure indigo. Black henna has a chance of being a mix rather than straight indigo. The mixes often contain chemicals and additives. Like henna, pure indigo is safe to use regularly, and you can use it on chemically treated hair or if you're pregnant.

For the most part, we'll be using henna and indigo in the same manner as if using henna only. But first you need to determine the color you want. The more indigo you use, the darker your hair will be. The more henna you go with, the redder it will be.

For instance, if you use equal parts of henna and indigo on gray hair, you'll have a medium reddish-brown. ⅓ henna to ⅔ indigo gives you dark brown, while ⅔ henna to ⅓ indigo results in a lighter reddish brown. Again, the only way to know your results is to do a strand test first.

To recap on the amount of herb used, you'll need a combined total of 100 grams henna and indigo for short hair, 200 - 300 grams for shoulder length hair, and 400 - 500 grams for longer hair. Just don't mix your dried herbs together to weigh it. These will be prepared separately. Also, keep in mind you can't freeze leftover indigo, so don't make extra for later.

Follow the directions for mixing henna 12 hours ahead of time. Right before use, add your desired amount of indigo to the henna and use some water to get the thick yogurt consistency. Mix this very, very well to avoid streaking. If you think you have dye resistant hair, you can add 1 teaspoon of salt for every 100 grams of indigo used. Allow the mixture to sit for 15 more minutes before use.

Use it just like you would for coloring with henna only, applying in sections right to the roots. Cover your head in plastic wrap or a snug shower cap, then leave it on your head for anywhere from one to six hours. (The longer it's on, the darker your hair will be.)

Rinse thoroughly. This technique also requires two or three days for the hair to oxidize and find its true color, so if there's a hint of blue, don't panic. That will settle.

Using Henna and Indigo for Black Hair

You can get black results on any hair type, and it works especially well on African hair. I've heard some blondes end up with a bluish cast, however. Since my hair isn't blonde, I can't test this one out for you. (I'd also look dreadful with black hair, no matter how much I may long for dark tresses!) So again, strand tests are important to make sure you're getting what you want.

To achieve a rich black shade, you have to henna your hair first. Indigo on its own will give you blue hair, and if that's what you're into, I won't tell you no. The Manga look might work for you. But for anyone desiring black hair, you'll need to do the henna treatment as described earlier.

Once you've done a henna application and your hair is rinsed and dried, it's time to start the indigo. Use the same amount of indigo as henna. If your hair required 300 grams of henna, for instance, use 300 grams of indigo. Just keep in mind you can't freeze the leftover indigo like you can with the henna.

If you think your hair is resistant to dyes, you can add a teaspoon of salt for every 100 grams of indigo you use. Mix the indigo powder with water until you get that thick yogurt consistency. You'll notice it seems a bit more like wet sand, however, so for ease of use you may add one or two eggs to the mix. Personally, I can't tolerate the smell of raw eggs on my head. Just a warning in case you're like me and don't want to get the gags. With or without the eggs, let the indigo sit for 15 minutes before use.

Apply the indigo just like you did with the henna, wrapping your hair with plastic wrap or a tight shower cap. Allow the indigo to stay on your hair for an hour or two, then rinse thoroughly.

It'll take two or three days for the hair to oxidize, so don't panic if you look a bit on the blue side. That should settle shortly. If you find you've missed a spot or something's uneven, feel free to mix up a bit more and apply it where needed. It won't hurt your hair.

Using Cassia for Blonde Hair

For those of you who insist blondes have more fun, perhaps you're feeling a bit left out at this point, what with all our talk about redheads, brunettes, and exotic raven blacks. Don't break out the tissues just yet — there's an herb for you, too, and it's called cassia.

Cassia obovata can actually be used on all hair colors, although it will only return golden hues for those with blonde, gray, or white hair. For the rest of us, however, it's a fantastic conditioner.

Cassia is prepared in much the same way as henna, and like henna, leftovers can be frozen for later use. Mix it with your choice of lemon or orange juice 12 hours before needed. Add enough juice to get it the consistency of thick yogurt; cover it with plastic and allow it to sit overnight. (Again, don't forget to do a strand test to make sure you get the color you want, and a skin test to check for allergic reactions.)

Apply the cassia to your hair in sections right to the scalp. Make sure it's on thick and that your hair is completely covered. Wrap your head in plastic wrap or a tight shower cap and allow it to sit for about three hours. Rinse thoroughly.

If you have a darker shade of hair and would like to use cassia as a conditioning treatment, allow it to sit on your hair for about an hour before rinsing thoroughly.

Strawberry Blonde Shades for Blonde and Gray Hair

If you have blonde, gray, or white hair, you can experiment going strawberry blonde by using 80% cassia with 20% henna. Use the mixture just like you would if you were using straight henna or cassia. Prepare 12 hours ahead of time, apply to hair in sections right to the scalp, and leave on wrapped hair for three hours before rinsing thoroughly. Again, strand test first, please! (Leftovers of this one can be stored in the freezer for later use.)

Natural Hair Lighteners

I remember back in the '80s, the big hair lightening rage was a product that you sprayed on your head and heated up with a blow dryer or the sun. Boy, did I love that stuff! I got the extra super-duper variety, since all 16-year-old girls understand that more is better, and tried to streak my hair with it. At some point in the application, combing it through seemed the "intelligent" course, and before I knew it, my medium brown hair was a bright (yet somewhat crispy) blonde.

Fortunately, I rolled with the results just fine. But back then, I wasn't hip on what makes for truly healthy hair, which doesn't include dumping bottles of chemicals onto my porous and thirsty scalp.

If you want to lighten your hair, there are a couple of interesting and very healthy options for you. One involves honey, the other lemon juice.

Let's start with the lemon juice since that's the easy one. Lemon conditions the hair and makes it soft and shiny. You can even make a hairspray from it (as shared in my book *Beauty Gone Wild! Herbal Recipes for Gorgeous Skin & Hair*). But if you want a good hair lightener, nothing could be easier.

Mix 2 tablespoons of lemon juice (natural, please — no plastic lemon squeezie stuff) with one cup of water and work it into your hair. Leave it on for about two hours while sitting in the sun, for best results.

If you'd like to give honey a try, it's not very difficult, either. Honey contains some natural hydrogen peroxide, and adding cardamom or cinnamon gives this effect a bit of a boost. You can do this repeatedly until you arrive at your desired shade. It can even add highlights to darker shades.

Just about any raw honey will work, although honeys with higher levels of vitamin C should be avoided. These would be honeys such as anzer, buckwheat, linden, locust, mint, and thyme.

Here's what you'll need:

raw honey
distilled water (1 Tbs. honey for every 6 Tbs. distilled water)
1 Tbs. ground cardamom or cinnamon (per cup of honey and water)
1 Tbs. extra virgin olive oil (per cup of honey and water)

Mix everything together very well, allow it to sit an hour before application, then apply it to damp hair using a comb or a brush to help you get it evenly distributed. Wrap your hair well in plastic wrap, then cover your head with a snug shower cap or a bathing cap so your hair stays wet. Leave it on for an hour, then wash it out well.

Don't try to use heat with this treatment. Using a blow dryer or sitting in the sun can ruin the peroxide in the honey.

Herbs for Temporary Color Rinses

If all that coloring seems like too much fuss for you but you still want some color, there are several herbs that offer various shades in the way of a rinse. For all the herbs below, prepare a strong tea and follow your regular hair washing by rinsing with a mug of herbal brew. Or pour the color repeatedly over your head while leaning over a bowl. The bowl will catch the tea which can then be poured over your head once again. This will speed up the process.

Remember, the resulting tint will depend largely on your hair now. So if you're concerned with the results, sacrifice a strand of hair for testing purposes. These are temporary colors and not drastic, so if you get a shade you don't like, have no fear. It will fade.

Herbs that Enhance Hair Color

Blondes & Light Shades: Chamomile, calendula (gives a reddish tint), lemon peel, mullein flowers

Brown Shades: Elderflower, birch bark, cloves, cinnamon chips

Brown and Black Shades: Black malva, sage, rosemary, black walnut hulls

Red Shades: Calendula, rose petals, beetroot powder (use a muslin tea bag when steeping), red hibiscus

Gray Shades: Sage, elderflower, lavender

Natural Styling Products

Your hair is free of commercial products. You've successfully given up shampoos, boxes of hair color, mousse, hairspray, gels... What? You don't want to give up styling your hair just because you gave up the chemicals? I do understand. For me, this was quite a hurdle too. I'll admit I wear a pretty simple hairstyle. And while going no 'poo definitely makes fixing my hair much easier, I do still like to use a bit of hairspray and styling product. But I don't buy the stuff. I make it. This is where we learn how.

Natural Hair Gels

If your hairstyle is more demanding and you can't part with hair gel, here's a quick tip. Try aloe. You can purchase 100% pure aloe vera gel online or in most health food stores. Just make sure what you get contains no additives or preservatives; most popular brands do! Use it just as you would any hair gel.

Flaxseed Hair Gel

Flax is wonderful for the hair, and this gel recipe incorporates its goodness. Of course, I'd recommend you eat flax for hair, skin, and overall health too! (One to two teaspoons a day of fresh ground flaxseed sprinkled on your food is all you need.)

For the hair gel, combine ¾ cup water and 1 tablespoon of whole flaxseed. Bring to a boil and allow the mixture to simmer for 15 minutes. Strain out the seeds and store it in the fridge. Toss and make fresh after a day or two.

Fenugreek Gel

Some say the maple syrup-like smell is delicious; others say it's more like a curry scent. Whether that's a fragrance you enjoy or not is up to you to decide, but if you've always wanted to bottle the aroma of the Waffle House, here's your chance. Blend 1 tablespoon of powdered fenugreek with hot water until the powder can no longer absorb more water. Apply to hair as a gel. Prepare as you need it. Serve with a side of hash browns and sausage links.

Old-Fashioned Hair Pomade

Hair pomades offer one way to style the hair and add a lustrous shine. It's especially good if you've got coarse hair. If you've not used one before, apply with restraint. Too much of a good thing is — well, no longer a good thing.

What You'll Need:

¼ cup sweet almond oil
5 drops bergamot essential oil
1 ounce beeswax, grated or pastilles

Place a medium saucepan on the stove filled about halfway with water. In a 1-cup measuring cup, place the sweet almond oil and the beeswax, then set them both in the pan. Heat slowly on low heat until all the wax is melted. Remove from heat, add the bergamot oil, and stir well. (I like wooden chopsticks.) Pour into a clean glass jar or balm container. When the pomade is completely cool, cap it tightly. Store it in a cool, dark place for a longer shelf life, anywhere from one to three years.

Old-Fashioned Hair Pomade #2

Not a very original name, but you can just call it #2 if you want to sound hip and in the know.

What You'll Need:

.8 ounces beeswax, grated or pastilles

15 ml. jojoba oil

1 Tbs. arrowroot powder

20 drops essential oil of choice

Fill a medium saucepan with water about halfway. Put beeswax into a 1-cup measuring cup and place it in the saucepan. Bring the water to a slow simmer, and allow the beeswax to melt completely. Turn the heat off and leave the measuring cup in the pan. Add the jojoba oil to the beeswax, stirring well so the two are completely mixed. Add the arrowroot powder and the essential oils and stir well. Carefully remove the hot measuring cup and pour the pomade into a clean glass container with a tight fitting lid for storage.

To use, take a pea sized amount and rub it between your fingers. This will warm and soften it, making it easier to work through your hair.

Boosting Your Hair's Potential

Got curly hair but you want it curlier? Want to control smooth, straight hair? Or maybe you're desiring an extra dose of shine. Even if you want to give your hair growth a kick in the pants, there's an herb for that.

A Secret to Incredibly Shiny Hair

If you want hair that really shines, you must get yourself a nice big bag of organic horsetail (*Equisetum arvense*). The herb horsetail contains silica and a host of minerals and goodness that make it just right for excellent hair health. It is important, however, to get organic when purchasing horsetail. This is an herb that grows waterside near rivers and streams, scooping up all the rich minerals and deposits from the water like a magnet. It's so good at this that when gold is present in a river, horsetail sucks it up too. But that also means that if it's growing downstream from a farm or a factory, it'll snag up all the pesticides and pollutants it can. So spend the extra couple of dollars and go for the organic version. It lasts a long time, and it's very much worth it.

You can prepare a hair rinse with horsetail by simmering about three tablespoons of dried herb with three or four cups of water for 15 minutes. Allow the tea to cool, then strain it well. Use it warm or cold as your final rinse. If you use it cold, your hair will be even shinier. No need to rinse it out, either.

You can drink the tea as well. There are lots of cautions floating out there on the web about the use of horsetail, claiming it will cause liver damage over time, but this is not entirely correct. If you eat the herb itself, yes, this may happen. (You won't want to — it's like chewy lawn clippings.) But if you drink the tea (organic, of course), you're fine. Also, make sure it's subspecies *Equisetum arvense*. If you're pregnant or nursing, there isn't enough research to tell if it's okay for you, so skip it until later. Also, don't buy horsetail in capsules to increase hair health. And dump out the herb you strained out of the tea. But you weren't going to eat that anyway, were you?

Remember, hair isn't actually alive. By the time it's grown from your scalp, it's dead material. Not that appealing to think about, I know. But the truth is, the only way to get really healthy hair is by what you put *in* you — not *on* you. Rinses improve the condition of what you've already got. A good diet is the only thing that can improve what you grow. We'll cover some more dietary ideas a bit later.

Detangler & Anti-Frizz Spritz

If you opted to go no 'poo, it's only a matter of time before tangles become a non-issue. I noticed mine disappeared within the first few days. But for curly or coarse hair types, frizz can still be an issue, especially on the humid or rainy days of summer. The following spritz recipe offers you a lightly fragrant anti-frizz remedy that will knock out any tangles along the way.

What You'll Need:

1 tsp. aloe vera gel (100% pure, no additives, etc.)
½ tsp. grapefruit seed extract (This acts as a natural preservative.)
2 drops grapefruit essential oil
2 drops glycerin (Not glycerin soap — just pure glycerin.)
8 oz. distilled water

Mix all the ingredients together and pour into a spray bottle. Spray it on freshly washed damp hair. Store it in your shower for ease of use.

Curl Intensifying Rinse

For an extra boost on the curls along with a healthy dose of shine, mix the juice of one lemon with 16 ounces of purified water. Use it as your final rinse, and don't rinse it back out. If this combination makes your hair feel a bit oily, cut back on the lemon juice next time around. A word of caution here: lemon juice may lighten your hair, especially if you're headed for the beach. Also, this is a good rinse for weekly use, not daily, because it may cause drying.

Gum Arabic Rosewater Rinse

An old remedy I discovered in an out-of-print beauty manual written around the turn of the 20th century offered this solution to bringing curls back to hair that's gone straight. You can easily purchase Gum Arabic at health food stores and online.

The recipe is simple. Combine 100 grams of Gum Arabic with 400 grams of rosewater. If you don't have access to rosewater, you can make a substitution of strong rosebud tea. Use this mixture as a final rinse after washing.

Sea Salt Hair Softener

Salt softens water, and we all know that. But it can soften your hair too. This softening spray combines the power of sea salt with bentonite clay, which as it turns out, is what most of the inexpensive cat litters are. But I'd recommend going with a bentonite clay you find packaged for human use. I have read of people using the cat litter variety, but there's no accounting for the quality of something that's been packaged for feline toilet usage.

What You'll Need:

3 Tbs. sea salt
1 cup 100% bentonite clay
water

Put the clay and salt in a bowl and add about 6 or 7 ounces of distilled water. Stir well with a fork until all the clay and salt have dissolved. It should be quite watery. Put the mixture into a spray bottle and spray it on dry hair. Saturate well, then wrap your hair in plastic wrap or a bathing cap and wait for 30 minutes before rinsing your hair.

Softening Coarse Hair

Yogurt is an excellent natural hair softener. If you have especially coarse hair, you'll want to try this one out. Just make sure you're using a good all-natural Greek style yogurt — not the fruit and corn syrup fat free watery soupy mess that sometimes passes as yogurt. To use, wash and towel dry your hair, then work a big glop of yogurt in. Let it stay in for 15 minutes before rinsing it back out. You may now yell "Opa!" and break a plate in celebration of great hair.

Catmint Hair Growth

Maybe Kitty knows the secret to luxurious fur lies in her cat toy. Catmint (*Nepeta cataria*) — or catnip if you must — promotes hair growth. Prepare a strong tea and use it as your final rinse, being sure to massage it into your scalp.

Hair Growth Oil

For a bit of a hair growth speeder-upper, this hair oil offers a wonderful scent that uplifts and relaxes simultaneously. Ah, the wonders of essential oils!

What You'll Need:

3 drops lavender essential oil

3 drops lemon essential oil

3 drops rosemary essential oil

3 drops cedarwood essential oil

3 drops thyme essential oil

⅛ cup jojoba oil

⅛ cup grapeseed oil

Blend all oils together in a tight-sealing container, preferably something amber or green. (Or store it in the dark.) Massage it into your scalp in the evening for three to five minutes. Wash out in the morning. You may want to cover your pillowcase to avoid possible staining.

Healthy Hair Summertime Conditioning Rinse

The following is a summertime treat for hair because it incorporates a couple of fresh leafy items you can gather outdoors. It's based on a Native American recipe, although I'm sure the ancients didn't use warm beer on their hair. But they did rely on plants for healthy locks, that's for certain. To learn how to properly identify the plants, use a plant guide or visit one of my favorite sites, Encyclopedia of Life (http://eol.org).

What You'll Need:

3 large Jerusalem artichoke or sunflower leaves, fresh
2 large plantain leaves (Not like the banana; like the weed. If gathered from your yard, make sure they've not been sprayed or fertilized in at least a year.)
1 quart cold purified water
1 Tbs. apple cider vinegar
4 ounces flat beer

Wash and bruise the leaves, then place them in a pot. Add the water, cover, and simmer on low heat for 10 minutes. Leaving the cover on and the leaves in, allow the water to cool for a good 30 minutes. Strain out the leaves and pour the decoction into a clean glass jar. Add the cider vinegar. You'll now have a beautiful green liquid which can be stored in the refrigerator for up to a week.

To use on your hair, take four ounces of the liquid and mix it with four ounces of flat warm beer. After washing and toweling your hair dry, pour it over your hair and don't rinse it out. The remaining decoction stored in your fridge can also be used as a toning face wash.

Food & Supplements for Strong Shiny Hair

Hair is grown from the inside out. Now, that's a surprise statement. But how often do we think on that? The hair we grow is a direct result of how we treat our bodies. A healthy diet and drinking plenty of water are key. If you already know you're eating plenty of fresh fruits and vegetables, and if you've got a diet rich in omega-3's, and if you shun high fructose corn syrup (I just shivered typing that), you can consider adding a few supplements to your diet to boost the hair health.

Seaweed

Seaweed, although not a big American favorite, is fantastically healthy. There are numerous forms of it, so if it seems totally foreign to your taste buds, I'm not suggesting you eat it raw straight from the ocean. Health food stores carry organic dried seaweed in powdered form that can be sprinkled on foods or added to smoothies. It's also available in capsule form, although it's good to acquire a taste for it. Your hair will shine with thanks.

Bee Pollen

Another supplement to try is bee pollen. It supports not only shiny, healthy hair but a healthy body. Its benefits are too numerous to mention here and would indeed require another book, to be sure. But before you start on it, you'll need to make sure you have no allergic reaction. Take a granule and allow it to melt completely under your tongue. If you experience no allergic reactions such as an itchy throat or watery eyes, put a few more under your tongue. Do this every day for three to five days, just to ensure there are no allergies. Slowly increase your intake to ¼ teaspoon more each day until you're taking a tablespoon of bee pollen daily. Getting to know all the benefits of bee pollen is definitely worth the effort!

Sesame

Sesame is an ancient hair and skin remedy. The Babylonians prized its ability to add to beauty. Halva, an addictive little dessert that combines ground sesame seed with honey, has long been eaten to give hair and skin a youthful vitality. The Chinese incorporate sesame into many of their foods. Sesame seeds are loaded with all kinds of minerals essential for healthy hair, such as copper, calcium, magnesium, zinc, and more. Try adding toasted sesame to stir fry or salads. Hummus contains tahini, which is really just the peanut butter of raw sesame seeds. I even make tahini myself by using a heavy duty blender to grind sesame seeds with a bit of water.

Chia

Another tiny seed that packs a healthy punch is chia. Yes, those little seeds that grow hair on terra cotta bulls so popular back in the 1970s. You can still buy those today, but it's easier to just go to the health food store and ask for a bag of chia. I promise they won't laugh at you! Chia is loaded with omega-3 acids, fiber, and protein. My 5-year-old loves it when I give him a little cup of chia to snack on. Sometimes we add them to smoothies or make a fabulous chocolate pudding, which isn't entirely healthy, but we all need a dose of chocolate now and then. Might as well make it good for us!

Since your next question is, "How do you make the pudding?" I might as well tell you. Just think of it as dessert for your hair.

Ingredients:

2 ½ cups milk or soy milk

½ cup chia seeds

6 Tbs. cocoa or carob powder

¼ cup raw sugar, agave, or natural sweetener

½ tsp. vanilla extract

a pinch of salt

Dump all these ingredients into a food processor or powerful blender. (I use a Vita-Mix, which does a great job.) Mix on high until very smooth. Pour the pudding into a glass bowl, cover, and refrigerate before serving. Hide it in the back because once the family knows it's there, they'll eat it all before you get any. Or so I've experienced...

Flax

You've probably heard the term "flaxen hair." It's true, those little flax seeds are soft, slippery little buggers. But I wonder if the phrase also comes from flax's ability to aid in the health of skin and hair. A fantastic source of fiber and omega-3's, flax can transform your skin and hair with regular use. Start slow on this one. If you decide to jump in and consume a tablespoon on your first day, you may not leave the bathroom the next! Like I said, it's an excellent source of fiber.

The best way to eat flax is to purchase it as whole seed, then grind it in a coffee grinder right before using it. We store our seeds in the freezer so the oils in the seeds don't have a chance to go rancid.

You can sprinkle ground flax seed on just about anything. Salads, oatmeal, in smoothies, etc. Or eat them whole. Just make sure to chew them well because the magic of the seed is inside, and swallowing them whole won't work. Start small — say ¼ teaspoon — and work your way up to one or two teaspoons a day.

More Hair Healthy Foods

If things like chia and seaweed seem a little off the wall to you, there are plenty of foods that provide hair nutrition that you may find a bit more familiar. Your body requires plenty of omega-3 acids to give you shining hair and to avoid a dry scalp. Protein is needed for strength and good hair growth, and vitamins A and C are required to produce the sebum so vital to healthy hair. Of course, there's also the calcium, the iron, the B vitamins, and so much more that all goes into growing those tresses. As you can see, putting your energy into growing healthy hair certainly won't go to waste. The worst thing that could happen would be improved overall health! So what can you add to the table? Glad you asked.

Salmon is a big one; it's so high in omega-3's and protein, as well as B-12 and iron. And Popeye had it right with the spinach. Any dark leafy greens, in fact, are vitally important. Experiment with others such as kale, chard, and dandelion. (Yes, dandelion! Ask anyone over 70 years old who grew up on a farm. They'll remember eating it in their youth, for sure.) Beans are an excellent choice for adding protein and omega-3's, not to mention a whole host of minerals. I'm talking the legumes, the refried beans, bean soup, baked beans, three bean salad, etc.

Just make sure that whatever you do, you get healthy, whole foods in your diet and avoid things like refined sugars and processed foods. I know it's easier said than done when you've got a lifetime of eating habits built up, but the important thing is to take it one step at a time and think about it from the perspective of adding things rather than denying yourself. After awhile, you'll be surprised at how much your diet has changed, not to mention your hair and your overall health!

Conclusion

Hello, Beautiful!

If you've made it this far and given the old heave ho to all those bottles and chemical concoctions, then congratulations! You've no doubt experienced some real changes in your hair. Whether you chose to add only a few natural homemade hair recipes to your daily regimen or you've done the big hair makeover and gone no 'poo, the journey will have been well worth it. You've eliminated chemicals; made real lifestyle changes. Congratulations! Now, go forth and be fabulous.

Other Books by Diane Kidman

Herbs Gone Wild! Ancient Remedies Turned Loose

Beauty Gone Wild! Herbal Recipes for Gorgeous Skin & Hair

Teas for Life: 101 Herbal Teas for Greater Health

Acknowledgements

Thanks to those who read the book over and over again; to those who weren't afraid to do strange things to their hair and go out in public like that, then tell me what happened; and to my family who not only tolerates living with a woman who says things like, "I've decided to throw away all our shampoo," but whose answer is always, "Okay."